I0390381

"WE ARE LIKE BUTTERFLIES WHO
FLUTTER FOR A DAY AND THINK IT IS
FOREVER"
CARL SAGAN

ISBN: 9781095227602

© 2019 by Aneet Patel, MD FACC

No part of this book may be reproduced or distributed in any way without permission of the author. All rights reserved.

Hearts of Men

Poems & Prose by
Aneet Patel, MD FACC

For Sarah
For Remy
For my family and my patients

*

For the lives we have lost
For the joy yet to follow

Contents

Preface

As we walk in this world one thing becomes clear
Time is the currency of this life
Slow then fast, fleeting in memory.
What other truths to follow you may know already
but in this book of poems and prose I find them again for
safekeeping in this world

BLIND

In moments of time

Periods of solace
Some with haste

Breathless for air
Our center
Our core

Trembling.
It knows, but cannot see
It feels but cannot see
The hearts of men

YOU AND I

You know that I can hurt too
I can hurt you
But I will do this thing
What hardest thoughts I have
What sorrow you bring
I hurt for you
I'll break my heart for you

But know that I may be broken too

Entrance

I've waited outside this door
Fellow traveler
From which side the waves come we do not know

A person behind, a person before
We grow weary as the day stretches before us
I know you will feel warmth from this
It may be fear or relief
I'll find you clarity in this
One voice to guide, the choices are yours
Our journey has just begun

EXIT

Life in a moment
The life in your eyes
What are you thinking?
I'm here, I won't leave you
I know I'll leave you

I'm sorry
I've cracked your chest
I've made you vomit
I don't ask before I do

Breathe

Don't breathe- please don't feel this
Please don't feel this
Don't see this.

FAITH

Trust is built
Trust is love
Trust is lost

We cannot do this without each other
But we have to face it alone.

THE MEND

Each moment of nourishment
Each smile
Each tear
Each laugh
Each quiet moment
Orders and codes damned

Units have no foot on the ground.

Units don't breathe easier in the night.

Units don't experience gratitude or fear or loss or gain.

Units were not made for us.

They were made for them.

A hand before us, strength in grip
Trust in me, see me.

No clocks are on the walls in here

only time will tell
What hearts will become

Pan positive

Fuck
I have no idea
Let's try this again in two weeks

Cycle

Emptied day to fill again

Fill me with love my son
Fill me with trust my love
Help these painful memories be lost with time
I'm sorry I cannot feel yours today

Fill my heart
Only so that I may pour it out again

Spectacles

One thousand points ahead
Three thousand points behind
Shadows and color
Sound passed where light does not
Light passes where sound cannot
Hear my gait
Know me
Tell me your story
Prey we are not outlasted

Brilliant

I'm not aware of the things that I know
Or when I learned of you

But I knew of your heart before

I've seen its soul beside
a ghost beneath

a quiet cage, the doors and it's walls
are aged but steadfast

Reconcile

Pills to bring you joy
Pills to clear the sorrow
Pills to test your courage
Pills to soften your swallow

Pills to quell your thirst
Pills to help you remember

Pills not given but taken by vein
Pills from doctors to follow

I pray my thoughts give you more time in this life
I pray they succeed more than others

I know they cannot replace the time that has passed
But time is not encapsulated with ease

Torn

I'm scared

                                        I know but I'm here.

I want to wait a few more weeks

                                        I will walk us through it.

I'm scared

                                        It's the only way.

Be brave dear friend
No time for goodbye.
Say anything of fear, it is real

                                        And it lingers with time

ACCESS

It's cold in here.
The floor is cold.
Thin robes, thick clogs, mesh and plastic
Lights above are blanched and bright
Lights above are never pointed just right
Skin and sweat
Aging stubbled chin
Echos of noise
Holes and tubes and blood and return
Bubbles beware
But don't be scared
Be afraid, be cautious as these moments count.

Don't fuck this up, Don't fuck this up. Don't rip. Don't push. Feel your
hands.

Don't fuck this up

They count for you and they count for him

My foot feels warm
Why is my foot warm?
Oh, its blood.

This time

Stay with me. Please, I cannot be alone doc
they've abandoned me here.

                    Few words, no discourse needed tonight
                               Is there enough time
                            Do the right thing he said
                         Enough time to drive back in
                    Scribbled edge--It's not good this time.
                    Thousands have passed before this one

                              Time to rouse the weary

I enter the numbers
I don't know what I'm going to say
I wake up his brother on the east coast
I don't know how to say it
I'm going to say it

Color of You

This doesn't define you
It doesn't define me
Words on a page
Voices heard
Voices echoed
It is the color of you today
But you are a painting
And I will give it a name

The word is strong
You have heard it before
It has more meaning than you know
I know it brings fear to your heart
We will mix all these colors together and change what it means
The fear will die if we change what it means

TEMPEST

You are lost in this ocean
Let's make this time count
What rations have you left
What strategies have we left

I'm lost with you
But I've studied the maps
I remember and have made the maps
I drew them until my mind could not bear witness again

I know waypoints are near
I feel they are near
Hold on

Ten minutes today
Fifteen next week
We are closer today, and further the next
Land is our dream
Water our reality
Rocking

The endless deep of uncertainty
This ocean will not forgive

Steady this ship
We have the surface on our side
This time only a thimble
Next time a bucket
Three times a day, two times a day, once a week
Forward

Salt and water crack your lips
Water will sink

Most of us make it
Some will not
But i'll be here
The tempest is yet to follow

QUESTIONS

How much light passes through you
How much light bounces back

Recreated

\\

Is your soul inside?

Who will answer

\\

And what does it hide

Attention

Quiet now
Listen for truth
Truth is abound

Quiet now
Listen for signs
What ebbs must flow
The center then left
What ripples and tides to find below

Quiet now
A flutter inside
Born smooth
Turned loud
No longer it seeks to relinquish and hide

Quiet now

Quiet

Story

Red numbers and arrows
Black numbers and arrows
Blue letters and arrows

This warm wind eddies
Pushing through the rift
Beating with force above the ridge
Coupled with time

Two exclamation marks
Numbers pile
Lists and dots
Phrases filled
Pictures pasted

The bell whistles
Pressure builds
Listen
See

How far from your truth is this mirror of you
This craft we build from word
Judgement of sight
Your texture, its heat
Recorded in time

It is my memory of you
The color of you I saw that day
A picture taken with words and digits
I see what you want me to see
And what you do not know of yourself

Red numbers and arrows

Black numbers and arrows
Blue letters and arrows
This record of you

If only it could come
And tell us stories in the night

Cadence

Dear friend
Repeated cadences
encountered
Repeated cadences
But not this one before

Dear friend
This sound remembered

Its cadence slow

In the deep from where this came-
such resolute sorrow

Dear friend
You need no permission from me

Your life is your story
Your life is your own
It has been long
But in this world its time is ending

I am what you ask of me
Dear friend

Orders

Steady line, black ink
Scratched in this paper
Written in words
This is my wish for you

Was it heard
Will it return for us
Promises kept or broken
Only with practice may wish be truth
The road paved now, from cobblestone and dirt and mud and forest
This is my wish for you

Twenty Two days

In the beginning
From form and structure
Twenty two days

Years spent for this moment
Seconds only spent living it
Your mother took pause
And we looked at eachother.

An invisible spark
Its energy in waves
Light in the dark

It grew, it stretched
It folded
It filled; awake
It beat
Within us and within you

Your heart
Our heart
Made whole again

ENEMY

I see your body frail
Weak from torment
Hungry for air
Hungry for forgiveness
It moves faster now

Where do we go from this place
We all go through this place

I'll find words with hope for you
I hope I'll find words with hope for you
I'll tell you it's alright

What silent monsters do you face
What lurks beneath
I've heard this one before

I see your body frail
Falling apart, forfeit
Not long now
We both know
We don't talk about it today

We don't have to because we both know

I'll find words with hope for you
I'll tell you it's alright
You already know it's alright

So today you ask

Where do we go from this place

GLOW

Your heart glows today
Collisions and ember not harmful but bright
Beacons that shine
From points in the dark
Beacons that shine
Not seen but heard

Through sinew and bone its rays will fly
Annihilations abound
Undeviated trajectory
Unrelieved
Uninterrupted

Flooded fields
Scintillating

Cool blues and specks, counts and statistics
A sea of orange made from crystal
Processed and remade again

Nothing could be closer to magic
This painting of you
Atom from atom

Truth not true
False not false

Your heart glows today
As if it did not already before

SQUEAK

The door inside of you narrows
It whistles, burning in my ear
It speaks but doesn't listen
Pressure

The door inside of you narrows
forced open to let your spirits pass

Rusted hinges
So many crossings
Wise but tired from so many crossings

Wandering now

You look the same
But you are different

Finite

The door inside of you narrows
Clock points to midnight

The door inside of you narrows
What do you choose
What to offer
A long night or mornings few

We have three doors to choose from
And we can do this on Tuesday

STRANGLED

It's not normal
I don't feel that I'm right inside
What is it
That you feel is not right inside

I've pushed and I've walked but the pressure keeps holding
I sweat like a river
My legs are unfolding

It's not normal
I don't feel alright inside
What is it that you feel is not right inside

DOUBLE A

I'm watched tonight
Silently watched
beside my dreams
Stirring from an age long lost

Messenger
What message does it bring
What message from the cold
From the blanched hallways that echo
quiet now but stirring

What alarm has rung
Slumber no more

I'm watched tonight
Rumbling messages
Distress

Restless I've grown from its call
Soothed the messenger
Aged the messaged
Silent watcher
Beside my dreams

Nocturnal

Dimming light
I've wandered these halls
Night after night
Shadows on these walls
Night after night

Laughter heard in the distance
Sadness in another
Is it my own

Fires crackle and jump
Not enough rain for each

Lists collected
Names forgotten
Faces remembered
Lives remembered

Days in slumber
Dreams of sun
Dreams of mountains

The world sleeps tonight
But hearts do not

The world sleeps tonight
But hearts do not

TURBULENT

Irresolute heart
Cooling; mottled now
Leaving this place
Heart like stone

Short distances now a journey

How heavy the blanket to choose
Too heavy and you'll drown
Too light and you'll suffer

In the forest your embers burn
Fed by the air of time

LETTERS

Letters of trust
Letters of thanks
Letters of heartache
My son, my father, my wife, my love.
Futures kept
Promises held
Never spoken

You see the one truth
Is to never promise
Is never to tell
But to guide
To partner
To follow through
Friend of reality

Letters of mine
Locked tight in memory
To spend on those lost
To spend when I'm lost
The few of many

With enough time and a bit of luck
If we see the signs right today
With a bit of luck
We are ready for tomorrow

TRUTH

I'm looking for a nice way to say this
Maybe truth is enough

Short seconds of pause

Breathe in
Breathe out

Left
RIght
Lower left
Lower right

Doors open
Passing dangers

I'm looking for a good way to say this
Maybe truth is enough
It's never enough

Everyday

My shoes are worn
My strength is worn
Alcohol stained
Broken laced
Holes in the socks but you cannot see
Buttons missed but you cannot see

Not enough time to think before I speak
On point today
Don't miss the details
Heart on fire
On point today
Mind like water

I have to be on point today
Everyday

The consequence is severe
Everyday

UNTIL TOMORROW

About the Author

Dr. Aneet Patel is a board certified cardiologist practicing in Seattle Washington. He was born in Alberta, Canada. His childhood was marked by international residences in Texas and Saudi Arabia and ultimately grew up in Peachtree City, Georgia. Dr. Patel graduated with a bachelor of science in microbiology and minor in social psychology at Georgia Tech. He completed his training in medical school at Emory University School of Medicine where he met his wife who is also a physician. After residency in Internal Medicine at the University of Washington in Seattle, he then completed his fellowship in cardiovascular diseases.. He is quadruple boarded in internal medicine, cardiology, echocardiography and nuclear cardiology.

As a prior clinical instructor at the University of Washington and medical director of cardiovascular imaging at The Polyclinic, he has been committed to providing excellence in patient care, teaching and serving as a mentor to the next generation of cardiologists as an active member of the American College of Cardiology.

He lives in Seattle with his wife and son where they enjoy travel, music, hiking, the outdoors, photography and spending time with each other.

www.ingramcontent.com/pod-product-compliance
Lightning Source LLC
Chambersburg PA
CBHW030737180526
45157CB00008BA/3205